DHEA FOR BEGINNERS

Unlocking Vitality, Harnessing The Power Of DHEA For Health, Impact On Hormonal Balance, Energy, Aging, Longevity, Maximizing Wellness And Performance

Georgette Lockett

DISCLAIMER

The author of this book is not affiliated, associated, endorsed, sponsored, or approved by any company or individual. The views and opinions expressed in this book are solely those of the author and do not necessarily reflect the official policy or position of any entity.

The author hereby disclaims any relationship, collaboration, or partnership with any company or individual mentioned in this book. Any references to products, services, or individuals are provided for informational purposes only and should not be construed as an endorsement or recommendation.

Readers are advised to exercise their own judgment and discretion when applying the information provided in this book. The author shall not be held responsible for any actions taken by readers based on the content of this book.

This book is intended for general informational purposes only, and the author makes no representations or warranties of any kind, express or implied, about the completeness, accuracy, reliability, suitability, or availability of the information contained herein. Any reliance on the information in this book is at the reader's own risk.

The author reserves the right to update, change, or modify any information in this book without notice. It is the responsibility of the reader to verify any information before taking any actions based on the content of this book.

By reading this book, the reader acknowledges and agrees to the terms of this disclaimer.

INTRODUCTION

DHEA is a precursor of many hormones, including testosterone and estrogen, and plays an important role in maintaining the body's hormonal milieu. DHEA has received attention as a naturally occurring hormone owing to its numerous physiological roles and possible health benefits.

This section tries to give a fundamental overview of DHEA, including its synthesis, functions, and significance in the human body. It lays the groundwork for a thorough examination of DHEA's mechanisms, uses, and prospective effects on health and wellbeing.

DHEA is predominantly generated in the adrenal glands and, to a lesser degree, in the gonads. It is an important precursor in the production of androgens and estrogens, which are the principal sex hormones. This hormone plays an important role in a variety of physiological functions, from immune function and metabolism to mood control and cardiovascular health.

The goal of this book is to dig extensively into the many facets of DHEA, investigating its biochemical routes, biological roles, prospective therapeutic uses, and the debates surrounding its supplementation. This guide seeks to give a full knowledge of DHEA's function in human health and well-being by analyzing its methods of action and varied impacts on the body.

This book tries to provide a complete understanding of DHEA, covering both its potential and limits in the realms of health and medicine via an examination of scientific research, historical context, and practical applications.

CHAPTER 1

Understanding DHEA

What Is DHEA?

Dehydroepiandrosterone (DHEA) is a steroid hormone generated predominantly by the adrenal glands, which are positioned directly above the kidneys. It is one of the most abundant hormones in the human body, acting as a precursor to both male and female sex hormones such as testosterone and estrogen. DHEA is essential for many physiological activities, contributing to general health and well-being.

Biological Functions And Role In The Body

DHEA is a versatile hormone that has many functions in the body:

1. DHEA is a precursor of androgens and estrogens, which are essential for the development and

maintenance of reproductive tissues as well as secondary sexual characteristics.

2. Immune Function: It has been proposed that DHEA has immunomodulatory effects, regulating immune system function and perhaps having a role in immunological responses.

3. Cognitive performance: Some research has looked at the link between DHEA levels and cognitive performance, suggesting that DHEA may have a role in memory and general brain health.

4. DHEA has been linked to bone metabolism, and appropriate amounts may aid in maintaining bone density and avoiding osteoporosis.

5. DHEA levels tend to fall with age, and some feel that supplementing with DHEA may help with energy and vitality, especially in those who are suffering age-related losses.

Production And Regulation

DHEA production occurs throughout puberty, peaks in the late teens to early twenties, and then declines with age. DHEA is mostly produced by the adrenal glands, although minor quantities may also be produced by the testes and ovaries.

DHEA synthesis is regulated by a complicated interaction of hormones, with pituitary adrenocorticotropic hormone (ACTH) prompting the adrenal glands to create DHEA. DHEA levels may be affected by factors such as stress, disease, and age, resulting in fluctuations in concentration in the body.

Understanding DHEA's physiological functioning and control is critical for comprehending its potential involvement in different facets of health and investigating its uses in medical and wellness settings.

CHAPTER 2

DHEA And Hormonal Balance

Relationship Between DHEA And Other Hormones

DHEA (dehydroepiandrosterone) is a steroid hormone that the adrenal glands, gonads, and brain create. As a precursor to many hormones in the body, it plays an important function in hormonal equilibrium. It is converted by enzymatic mechanisms in many tissues, resulting in the creation of androgens, estrogens, and other hormones.

Impact On Testosterone And Estrogen Levels

DHEA has a substantial impact on hormonal balance. It is both a precursor to testosterone and estrogen. DHEA may be turned into testosterone in men, adding to the androgen pool.

In females, DHEA may be converted into estrogen, which helps to maintain hormonal balance and supports a variety of physiological processes.

Role In Reproductive Health

DHEA levels are linked to reproductive health in both men and women. DHEA levels that are adequate are associated with optimal sexual function, fertility, and desire. DHEA conversion to testosterone helps males maintain reproductive health, while estrogen production helps women maintain monthly regularity and general reproductive well-being.

However, it is important to highlight that DHEA's involvement in reproductive health is complex and requires a delicate hormonal balance. DHEA levels that are too high or too low might upset this equilibrium, thereby affecting fertility, sexual function, and reproductive cycles.

Understanding the interdependence between DHEA and other hormones is crucial to understanding its function in maintaining overall hormonal homeostasis inside the body. Any changes in DHEA levels have the potential to disrupt the delicate balance of several hormones, affecting a variety of physiological processes.

CHAPTER 3

DHEA And Aging

Effects Of Aging On DHEA Levels

Individuals' bodies endure a variety of hormonal changes as they age, including a decrease in DHEA (dehydroepiandrosterone) synthesis. DHEA is largely produced by the adrenal glands and serves as a precursor to many hormones, including testosterone and estrogen. DHEA levels begin to fall gradually around the age of 30, becoming more pronounced as one gets older.

Potential Benefits For Age-Related Issues

1. DHEA may have a role in promoting cognitive function, according to certain studies. Its reduction has been linked to age-related cognitive decline, and research is continuing to see whether

supplementation might improve cognitive capacities in the elderly.

2. DHEA has been related to improved bone health. It has been found in studies to help preserve bone density and reduce the risk of osteoporosis, particularly in postmenopausal women.

3. Immune System: DHEA has immunomodulatory effects and is thought to have a function in immune system maintenance. Its loss with age may have an impact on immune function, and several research are looking at its involvement in boosting immunological responses in older persons.

4. DHEA may alter muscular strength and metabolism, possibly supporting muscle function and overall energy levels as people age.

DHEA Supplementation In Older Adults

Because endogenous DHEA levels fall with age, there has been interest in supplementing DHEA to possibly reverse some of the impacts of aging.

The use of DHEA supplements in older persons, on the other hand, is a source of contention and current study.

1. **Individual Variability:** DHEA supplementation may have varied effects on different people. Before beginning supplementation, consider factors such as current hormone levels, general health, and particular medical issues.

2. While some studies show possible advantages, the long-term effects and safety of DHEA supplementation, particularly in elderly populations, are currently being studied. Potential negative effects and drug interactions should be carefully examined.

3. **Consultation and monitoring:** Consultation with healthcare specialists is essential for older persons seeking DHEA supplementation. Regular monitoring and supervision are required to evaluate the effects and assure safety, particularly in light of possible hormonal effects.

Understanding DHEA's involvement in the aging process is complicated, and its supplementation for age-related disorders needs further research. The potential advantages must be balanced against the hazards, and continuing research seeks to clarify its function in promoting health and well-being in older persons.

CHAPTER 4

Psychological And Cognitive Aspects Of DHEA

Influence On Mood And Mental Health

DHEA, a precursor to both estrogen and testosterone, is important in mood control and general mental health. Several studies have shown that it may help with depression and anxiety symptoms.

DHEA has been linked to feelings of well-being, and its levels are often shown to be inversely connected to stress and mood disorders.

Higher DHEA levels have been associated with enhanced emotional balance, a more pleasant mood, and fewer incidences of depressive symptoms.

Cognitive Effects And Potential Implications

DHEA has been studied for its possible cognitive benefits, namely on memory, attention, and general cognitive performance. DHEA supplementation may improve specific areas of cognition, such as verbal memory and executive function, according to some studies. These results have piqued the curiosity of researchers interested in investigating its potential uses in age-related cognitive decline and neurodegenerative illnesses. However, further research is required to produce solid proof.

DHEA And Stress Management

The stress response system of the body is deeply associated with the hormone DHEA. It acts as a counter-balancing hormone to cortisol, a stress hormone. DHEA and cortisol often function in opposition, and maintaining a balanced ratio of these hormones is critical for optimal stress management. The capacity of DHEA to alter the stress response has piqued researchers' curiosity in its potential as a stress-management treatment. However, further study is needed to determine the specific processes and efficacy in stress reduction.

DHEA's diverse involvement in mood, cognition, and stress response shows its potential as a mental health modulator. While early research suggests that it may be useful in treating mood disorders, enhancing cognitive function, and regulating stress, more well-controlled trials are needed to confirm its usefulness and safety in these areas.

Understanding DHEA's influence on psychological and cognitive elements not only gives insight into its possible therapeutic uses but also highlights the need for more study to investigate its specific mechanisms of action and appropriate dosage recommendations.

CHAPTER 5

DHEA And Physical Performance

Impact On Muscle Strength And Endurance

DHEA, a precursor to both estrogen and testosterone, has a function in muscle growth and maintenance. DHEA may increase muscular strength by increasing muscle protein synthesis and decreasing protein breakdown, according to research. It's thought to promote muscular development and help preserve muscle mass, especially in older people whose DHEA levels gradually fall.

Effects On Exercise And Athletic Performance

Athletes and fitness enthusiasts are often interested in drugs that may improve performance. Some studies have looked at DHEA's effect on exercise capacity and sports performance. However, results have been varied, with some research indicating possible benefits in muscular strength and power production while others showing no impact. It's important to remember that the benefits of DHEA on physical performance might differ depending on characteristics including age, gender, and baseline DHEA levels.

DHEA In Sports And Fitness

The usage of DHEA as a performance-enhancing substance has gotten a lot of interest in the sports world. DHEA supplements have been used by certain athletes and bodybuilders in the hopes of increasing muscular strength, decreasing body fat, and boosting overall athletic performance. However, because of possible health hazards and concerns about fairness in competitive sports, regulatory authorities often monitor and control the use of such supplements.

The effectiveness of DHEA supplementation in boosting physical performance is still being studied and debated. While some studies show possible advantages, the data is not conclusive, and a more extensive study is required to completely understand DHEA's influence on athletic performance.

It is important to emphasize that DHEA supplementation should be addressed with caution, particularly in the context of sports, since legislation and norms for its usage vary across various athletic organizations and governing bodies. Individual reactions to DHEA supplements may also differ, and any adverse effects or combinations with other drugs should be evaluated before usage. Before incorporating DHEA or any new substance into an athlete's routine, a healthcare practitioner or sports medicine specialist should be consulted.

CHAPTER 6

Health Conditions And DHEA

DHEA In Managing Specific Health Conditions

DHEA's role in the management of different health disorders is extensive. DHEA supplementation may augment hormone replacement treatment in disorders such as adrenal insufficiency or Addison's disease when the body fails to manufacture enough hormones. Furthermore, research is being conducted to investigate its potential in bone health disorders such as osteoporosis, since DHEA has been associated with bone density maintenance.

Potential Therapeutic Applications

Some research suggests that DHEA supplementation may provide therapeutic assistance in disorders such as depression, where those with reduced DHEA levels are more likely to experience depressed symptoms. Because of its ability to reduce pain and improve exhaustion, it is also being researched in chronic fatigue syndrome, lupus, and fibromyalgia.

Research On DHEA'S Role In Diseases

Research on DHEA's role in disease is ongoing. Because of its immunomodulatory qualities, various studies are looking at its potential in autoimmune disorders including multiple sclerosis and rheumatoid arthritis. Furthermore, its effect on metabolic syndrome, obesity, and insulin sensitivity is still being studied, since DHEA may alter glucose control and metabolism.

However, although studies indicate possible advantages, the use of DHEA as a medicinal agent is not widely approved or advised for any of these disorders.

The effectiveness and safety profiles differ, and further study is required before definite recommendations can be made.

DHEA has a wide range of effects, and continuing study tries to understand its function in a variety of health disorders. Understanding its mechanics and prospective uses may open up new possibilities for controlling and treating various illnesses.

CHAPTER 7

Safety And Side Effects Of DHEA

Potential Risks And Precautions

DHEA (Dehydroepiandrosterone) is a hormone naturally generated by the body's adrenal glands, and supplementing with it may have numerous implications and risks:

• **Hormonal Imbalance:** DHEA supplementation may boost androgen and estrogen levels in the body. This may upset the delicate hormonal balance and cause a variety of negative effects, particularly in those who already have hormonal disorders.

• **Effect on Other Hormones:** DHEA supplementation may affect the synthesis and balance of other hormones such as testosterone and estrogen. This shift may cause changes in mood, libido, and even metabolic functioning.

• **Unpleasant responses:** Some people may have unpleasant responses such as acne, hair loss, greasy skin, and changes in menstrual cycles (for women). These negative effects are associated with the androgenic effects of higher hormone levels.

• **Cardiovascular Effects:** Elevated DHEA levels may influence lipid metabolism and cholesterol levels, which may affect cardiovascular health in certain people. Those seeking DHEA supplements may need to monitor their cholesterol levels.

Adverse Effects And Contraindications

• **Psychological Effects:** DHEA can impact mood and behavior. While some people may feel better mood, others may suffer increased irritation, aggression, or mood fluctuations.

• **Drug Interactions:** DHEA may interact with drugs such as hormonal treatments, insulin, and corticosteroids, changing their efficacy.

If you're on any drugs, you should talk to your doctor before using DHEA.

Individuals with hormone-sensitive illnesses such as breast, uterine, or prostate cancer, as well as those with liver issues, diabetes, or other endocrine disorders, should avoid DHEA supplementation without medical supervision owing to the potential for deleterious consequences.

Safety Guidelines For Supplementation

• **Consultation with Healthcare Providers:** It is critical to consult with a healthcare practitioner before beginning DHEA supplementation, particularly if you have pre-existing health concerns or are using drugs. A doctor can determine if DHEA supplementation is safe and effective.

• **Dosage Control:** It is critical to follow the appropriate doses. Excessive DHEA use might result in more severe side effects and health hazards.

• Periodic monitoring of hormone levels, notably testosterone and estrogen, as well as lipid profiles, is recommended while taking DHEA supplements. This helps to ensure that levels remain within a healthy range and that any negative effects are minimized.

In conclusion, although DHEA supplementation may have some advantages, it is important to proceed with caution. Consultation with medical specialists and frequent monitoring are critical measures in mitigating possible dangers and ensuring safe use.

CHAPTER 8

Forms And Dosage Of DHEA

DHEA, or dehydroepiandrosterone, is a hormone that the body produces naturally, predominantly in the adrenal glands, with minor quantities produced in the gonads and brain. It is important in a variety of physiological processes since it is a precursor to other hormones such as estrogen and testosterone. When contemplating DHEA supplementation, it is critical to understand its types, doses, and absorption aspects.

Available Forms (Pills, Creams, Etc.)

DHEA Supplements are available in a variety of formats, including pills, capsules, sublingual tablets, and lotions. Each form has a different absorption rate and bioavailability. The most prevalent are oral tablets and capsules, which enter the digestive system before being absorbed. Sublingual pills dissolve beneath the tongue, allowing for direct absorption into the circulation and perhaps faster results. Topically applied creams skip the digestive system, offering a new pathway for absorption.

Recommended Dosage And Administration

DHEA dose varies greatly depending on parameters such as age, gender, health condition, and individual demands. Typical doses vary from 25 to 100 mg per day, while some people may need more or less. Experts often advise beginning with a smaller dosage and gradually increasing it while attentively watching how the body reacts.

The time of intake is also important. Some individuals choose to take DHEA supplements first thing in the morning to replicate the body's natural synthesis, while others spread the dose throughout the day to maintain stable levels.

Factors Affecting DHEA Absorption

Several variables determine how successfully the body absorbs and uses DHEA:

1. Route of Administration: The way DHEA is eaten affects absorption. Because they skip the digestive system, sublingual pills and creams may have higher absorption rates than oral supplements.

2. Individual Physiology: Age, metabolism, general health, and heredity may all influence how well the body absorbs and uses DHEA.

3. Other drugs or Supplements: Some drugs or supplements may interfere with DHEA absorption or efficacy. Before mixing DHEA with other drugs or supplements, it is critical to contact a healthcare expert.

4. Food and Lifestyle: Eating habits, food composition, and certain lifestyle variables may all have an impact on the body's capacity to absorb and use DHEA.

Understanding these distinctions enables people to make educated choices regarding the type, dose, and timing of DHEA supplementation, guaranteeing maximum absorption and efficacy while reducing possible dangers. Before beginning any supplementation plan, consult with a healthcare expert to identify the right dose and form based on individual health requirements and concerns.

CHAPTER 9

DHEA In Research And Clinical Trials

Overview Of Scientific Studies

Because of its potential impact on numerous areas of health, DHEA has received a lot of interest in scientific studies. Its effect on hormone balance, aging, mental health, and other factors has been studied. The initial emphasis of the study was on its impact on age-related disorders, but its scope has broadened to include wider health concerns.

Emerging Research Areas

Early research focused on the fall in DHEA levels with age and its possible link to age-related disorders. Several studies looked at whether DHEA supplementation may reverse some of these consequences, such as muscle mass loss, bone density loss, and changes in cognitive function.

Hormonal Imbalances And Health

DHEA has been studied for its function in resolving hormonal imbalances, particularly in diseases such as adrenal insufficiency or specific illnesses influencing hormone production. Studies have looked at its potential for treating several diseases, with a focus on restoring hormonal balance.

Mental Health And Cognitive Function

There is continuous research into how DHEA affects mental health and cognitive function. Its potential impacts on mood disorders, cognitive decline, and stress management have all been studied. Although some studies reveal a possible relationship between DHEA levels and mental health, a more thorough study is required.

Emerging Research Areas

Future research will explore further into DHEA's varied impacts and processes. Emerging areas of study include its possible involvement in metabolic health, its effect on immunological function, and research into its impact on particular disorders like as osteoporosis and autoimmune problems.

Obesity And Metabolic Health

Some research shows a possible relationship between DHEA levels and metabolic health, especially in diseases such as obesity or insulin sensitivity. DHEA is being studied to see how it affects metabolism and if it might be used to treat metabolic diseases.

Immunological Function

Preliminary study suggests that DHEA influences immunological responses and may have a role in immune function modulation. Understanding its effect on immunity may pave the way for further research into its therapeutic potential in immune-related illnesses.

Researchers are also investigating DHEA's impact on disorders such as osteoporosis, inflammatory diseases, and potentially some malignancies. The goal of these studies is to see whether DHEA supplementation may help with the development or treatment of certain illnesses.

Future Prospects And Ongoing Studies

The future of the DHEA study seems promising in terms of elucidating its multiple functions in health and illness. Ongoing clinical trials and research are looking at many elements of DHEA, such as optimum doses, possible adverse effects, and therapeutic uses in diverse populations.

Clinical Studies

To verify early results and establish the safety and effectiveness of DHEA supplementation, rigorous clinical studies are required. These studies include a wide range of cohorts and try to give more definitive data about the benefits and possible hazards.

Personalized Medicine And Hormone Therapy

As the area of personalized medicine evolves, there is increasing interest in understanding how DHEA supplements may fit into specialized treatment programs for people with unique health issues or hormone imbalances.

In conclusion, although early evidence suggests that DHEA has potential advantages, further study is needed to establish its function in clinical practice and determine its long-term impacts across multiple health domains.

Continued study will very certainly illuminate its methods of action and expand our knowledge of its therapeutic potential.

CHAPTER 10

Integrating DHEA Into Health And Lifestyle

DHEA (dehydroepiandrosterone) has received attention for its possible influence on several areas of health, perhaps providing advantages to certain people. Integrating DHEA into one's health and lifestyle involves careful assessment of its effects, possible advantages, and safety concerns.

Practical Applications In Daily Life

1. **Considerations for Supplementation:** DHEA supplements are available in a variety of forms, including tablets, capsules, lotions, and sublingual formulations. It is critical to understand the distinctions between these forms, as well as their bioavailability and delivery strategies.

2. **Consultation with Healthcare Providers:** Before integrating DHEA, it is critical to consult with a

healthcare practitioner. Individual health states, existing medicines, and possible interactions must all be discussed for informed decision-making.

3. Personal Health goals: It is important to recognize personal health goals. DHEA may be explored for age-related decline, hormonal imbalances, mood swings, or cognitive difficulties. Understanding how DHEA may connect with these goals is critical.

4. Monitoring and tracking: Regular health monitoring is recommended when taking DHEA. This involves keeping note of any changes in mood, energy, cognitive function, and hormonal balance.

Considerations For Using DHEA Supplements

1. Dosage and timing: It is critical to follow the suggested doses. Individuals may react differently to DHEA, thus it is normal, to begin with lower dosages and gradually increase them.

The timing of ingestion and knowing its half-life are other important considerations.

2. Potential Side Effects and Adverse Reactions: It is important to be aware of potential side effects such as acne, hair loss, changes in libido, and hormone imbalances. It is critical to monitor for any bad effects and seek medical help as soon as possible in such circumstances.

3. Long-Term Use and Cycles: DHEA supplementation is often done in cycles with intervals in between to minimize tolerance accumulation and to analyze the body's reaction.

DHEA As Part Of A Holistic Health Approach

1. Consider Lifestyle issues: Integrating DHEA into a holistic approach to health entails taking into account lifestyle issues. Nutrition, exercise, stress management, appropriate sleep, and general health habits are all part of this.

2. Complementary treatments: It is critical to understand how DHEA fits with other complementary treatments or supplements. It is critical to prevent possible interactions or effect duplications.

3. Continuous Assessment: It is critical to review the need for DHEA regularly within the context of an individual's health journey. Adjustments depending on changing health conditions or lifestyle changes may be required.

To summarize, incorporating DHEA into one's health and lifestyle takes careful thought, interaction with healthcare specialists, and knowledge of its possible benefits and drawbacks. It should be part of a complete wellness strategy that emphasizes individual health objectives and frequent monitoring for best results.

Conclusion

Throughout this book, we've looked at the many functions and consequences of DHEA in human health. DHEA has emerged as a crucial actor in a variety of physiological processes, from its fundamental definition to its critical influence on hormonal balance, aging, cognition, and beyond.

Understanding DHEA has revealed its deep linkages within the hormonal landscape, allowing us to watch its effect on testosterone, estrogen, and the delicate balance required for reproductive health and general well-being.

Aging has been a key area, with a focus on the possible advantages of supplements in treating age-related disorders and their consequences for mental clarity, mood control, and stress management.

However, DHEA's story goes beyond its possible advantages. We've gone over safety concerns, recognized the intricate interaction between supplementing and possible hazards, and emphasized the significance of following recommendations and consulting with healthcare specialists.

Exploration of various forms and doses, as well as current research and clinical trials, offers a picture of developing knowledge and an ever-expanding frontier of options for harnessing DHEA's potential.

We evaluated DHEA's practical uses and emphasized the need for a comprehensive approach when incorporating it into health and lifestyle activities. Understanding DHEA not only as a supplement but as part of a larger lifestyle story stresses its function within a holistic health paradigm.

As we get to the end of our journey, it's clear that DHEA sits at the intersection of science, health, and human physiology. Its importance stems not only from its recognized functions but also from the potential for future advancements, opening the way for more study and discoveries in the quest for human health and well-being.

While the tale of DHEA is still unfolding, it is an important chapter in understanding the inner workings of the human body and its role in leading a better, more balanced life.

This book is but a glimpse of the enormous terrain that DHEA traverses, and it is an invitation to continue investigating the delicate interaction between hormones and health, always with a focus on holistic well-being in mind.

THE END